Eat Smart, Burn Fat:

Revitalize Your Metabolism for Longevity.

By

Dr Albert M. Brose

Disclaimer page.

Welcome to 'Eat Smart, Burn Fat: Revitalize Your Metabolism for Longevity'! As you read through these pages, remember that there is a surprise at the conclusion of this book—a Free Gift to help you on your health journey even further. Thank you for coming on this transforming journey with us!"

Table of contents.

Introduction:

Calm Down Your Inner Flame - Discover the Keys to Metabolic Well-being and Extended Life.

Have you ever experienced a slowdown in your metabolism? Even when you work out regularly and monitor your diet, the weight doesn't seem to want to go away. You start to become frustrated and start to question whether having a faster metabolism is actually a hoax.

What if I told you that you can achieve metabolic health? It has nothing to do with strict workout regimens or trendy diets. It all comes down to realizing the amazing potential your body possesses and utilizing it to burn fat naturally.

The key to discovering the mysteries of metabolic health is this book, "Eat Smart, Burn Fat: Revitalize Your Metabolism for Longevity." Together, we'll set out on a life-changing adventure that will dispel falsehoods, breakthrough weight loss barriers, and rekindle your inner fire.

Your guide will be renowned metabolism and nutrition expert Dr. Albert M. Brose. Using the most recent findings from science and useful techniques, you'll learn:

The true story behind metabolism: We'll explain what metabolism actually is, what influences it, and why it's not necessarily the bad guy that people think it is.

The Eat Smart strategy: Ignore tight diet plans! We'll look at a cutting-edge diet that satisfies your hunger, speeds up your metabolism, and gives you a constant sense of energy.

The power of macronutrients: Discover how to use the energy of fats, proteins, and carbohydrates to build a customized diet that will assist your weight reduction objectives while nourishing your body.

Workout for metabolic transformation: Find out how to increase metabolism and shape a leaner, healthier body with weight training and smart cardio.

The often-overlooked elements like sleep, stress reduction, and hydration will be discussed as the "secret weapons of weight loss" and how important they are to reaching and maintaining a healthy weight.

This book provides a plan for a lively, healthy life rather than merely a weight loss manual. We'll provide you the information and resources you need to not just lose weight but maintain it off, feeling in control and energized all along the way.

Are you prepared to let go of your annoyance and move toward a future of energy and metabolic health? Now let's get started!

Chapter 1: Introduction: What Is Metabolism and Why Is It Important?

Think of your body as an amazing power plant that is always bustling with activity. Your metabolism is an internal powerhouse that controls everything from heart rate regulation to providing energy for everyday activities. However, your power plant is considerably more complex and exciting than a conventional one. It does more than simply provide energy—it changes the food you eat into the fundamental components of life!

Imagine a succulent, flavorful steak. The protein is broken down by your metabolism into amino acids, which are the building blocks of your muscles, organs, and even hair. It breaks down carbs into glucose, the energy source that keeps your brain functioning at peak efficiency. Even fat is important since it supports the generation of essential hormones and offers long-lasting energy.

However, metabolism does more than only convert food into energy. It's an ongoing delicate balancing effort that carefully controls your body's temperature, blood sugar, and even your mood. It is the quiet director of the symphony inside you, making sure that every instrument—your tissues, organs, and systems—is performing in unison.

Why then is this relevant?

Well, the cornerstone of a bright, active existence is a healthy metabolism. It's the reason you can dance all night long with a grin on your face and climb a mountain without getting tired. It supports a stronger immune system, aids in injury healing, and helps you keep a healthy weight.

What transpires, then, when things go wrong?

If your metabolism is slowing down, you may also experience persistent fatigue, low energy, and even struggle with uncontrollably gaining weight. You may have mood swings, sleep disturbances, or even an increased chance of developing long-term health issues.

Your guide to discovering the mysteries of your metabolism is this book. We'll dispel popular misconceptions, examine the science underlying this amazing procedure, and identify the critical elements that affect its effectiveness. More significantly, we'll provide you with the information and resources you need to maximize your metabolism and realize its full potential for a more vibrant, healthy version of yourself.

Prepare to:

Learn about the intricate world of metabolism and how it functions.

Find out the unexpected elements that might affect your metabolism.

Determine the underlying reasons for a slow metabolism that may be impeding your attempts to lose weight.

The path to a healthy you and a revitalized metabolism begins right now! Together, let's embrace your inner power plant and flip the page!

Opening the Internal Powerhouse

Picture your body as a beautiful, energetic metropolis that is ablaze with activity. For any structure or roadway to operate, energy must always flow through it. The food we consume provides us with this energy, which powers our metropolis. However, how does this food become the force behind our thoughts, actions, and heartbeats? Let us delve into the captivating realm of metabolism, the complex jigsaw of chemical processes occurring inside every one of our cells.

We're going to take a fantastic trip to investigate this metabolic powerhouse's inner workings in this chapter. We'll unlock the mystery of how a juicy burger may provide you with energy for your morning run or a bit of cake can help you stay focused on your next major project.

Get ready to be amazed as we explore:

The Metabolic Symphony: From the enzymes that lead the processes to the mitochondria that provide energy, we'll dissect the main members of this metabolic symphony.

From Food to Fuel: We'll walk you through the fascinating process by which food is converted into useful energy, from digestion to absorption.

The burning question: An explanation of burning calories that will help you comprehend how your body uses this energy for anything from developing muscle to keeping warm.

However, metabolism is more than just a mechanism for burning calories.

Metabolism is also very important for:

Creating a Stronger You: Discover how your metabolism contributes to the growth and repair of tissues, maintaining a robust and healthy body.

The Hormone Highway: We'll look at how your hormones and metabolism work together to affect everything from mood to weight control.

The Lifespan Connection: Learn about the unexpected relationship between metabolism and life expectancy and how knowledge of it may help one have a long, healthy life.

This chapter is about empowerment more than just science. Gaining insight into your metabolism's inner workings will enable you to maximize its potential and long-term health benefits. So fasten your seatbelts and get ready for an enlightening and thrilling journey into the inner realm!

Factors Affecting Metabolism: Uncovering Your Body's Internal Heat-Burning Engine

Ever wished you could regulate the rate at which your body burns calories? You can, which is wonderful news! The process of metabolism, which powers your energy and functioning, is dynamic. It's a complicated dance driven by an unexpected array of circumstances, and the secret to maximizing your body's capacity to burn fat is knowing these aspects.

Think of your metabolic process as a furnace. It requires the proper fuel (meal) and air (oxygen) to burn properly, much like a real furnace. Still, that's not all! The amount of heat that a fire burns depends on a number of factors, including the size and nature of the furnace (muscle mass), hormone levels, and environmental factors like the outside temperature.

Let's fuel the flames! The following are some of the major variables affecting your metabolism:

Muscle Mass: Even while at rest, muscle consumes calories since it is metabolically active tissue. Your basal metabolic rate (BMR), or the amount of calories your body burns merely to stay alive, increases with muscle mass. Gaining muscle with strength training is similar to fueling a fire with additional logs to keep it blazing hotter for longer.

Diet: Your metabolism is greatly influenced by the foods you eat. Because protein has a larger thermic impact than fat or carbohydrates, digesting it causes your body to expend more calories. Selecting complex carbs over refined ones aids in blood sugar regulation and helps avoid crashes that might impair your metabolism. Furthermore, hormone function, which affects metabolism, depends on proper lipids. Therefore, give up on fad diets and concentrate on providing your body with the proper nutrition.

Exercise: Getting your body moving will help you increase your metabolism. While cardio exercises burn calories while exercising, strength training produces a longer-lasting impact. Even at rest, your BMR rises when you gain muscle. Consider it as an afterburner for your furnace, allowing it to continue to burn hot long after your workout is over.

Sleep: Lack of sleep causes your body to create less leptin, the satiety hormone, and more ghrelin, the hunger hormone. Overeating and increased cravings may result from this, which may have a detrimental effect on your metabolism. It's similar to giving your furnace a tune-up to make sure it functions smoothly and effectively when you get enough good sleep.

Stress: Prolonged stress causes havoc with your hormones, especially cortisol, which can slow down your metabolism and cause you to gain weight. Acquiring knowledge about stress-reduction methods such as yoga or meditation can help you maintain healthy cortisol levels and a fast metabolism.

Through comprehension of these elements and implementing constructive modifications to your way of living, you may accelerate your metabolism and discover a more robust, youthful version of yourself. Recall that there are no miracle drugs or fast solutions. It all comes down to creating long-lasting routines that enhance your body's innate capacity to burn fat and maintain optimal health!

Chapter 2: The Myth of Slow Metabolism: Why There Could Be Fire Coming From Inside You

Let Go of the Blame Game: Exposing the Reality of Weight Gain, Has there ever been a moment when you thought staring at a piece of cake would make you gain weight? Do hours spent on the treadmill and countless salads appear to be producing little to no results? If so, you have probably heard about a sluggish metabolism in several weight reduction discussions as the cause. What if we told you, though, that this "slow metabolism" might not be real?

This chapter dispels the myth that weight gain is exclusively caused by a slow metabolism. We'll explore the intriguing science of your body's internal furnace and uncover the startling reality.

Exposing the Myth of Metabolism:

Debunked: We'll clarify what your metabolism is and isn't, as well as debunk the misconception that some individuals are just "born with a slow one."

Beyond the Basal Rate: This book will teach you about the unspoken variables that affect your metabolism in addition to your basal metabolic rate (BMR).

The True Causes of Weight Gain: We'll reveal the actual factors that might undermine your attempts to lose weight and leave you feeling angry.

Excuses, Not Empowerment:

This is not a chapter on assigning responsibility. It's all about arming yourself with information. You will discover:

How to Determine the True Cause of Your Weight Gain: Whether it's covert hormone imbalances, bad sleeping patterns, or cunning food sabotage, we'll provide you with the resources to determine the real causes of your weight gain.

Changing the Focus: We'll help you go from thinking about how to "fix my slow metabolism" to taking a proactive stance that is centered on improving your metabolic health.

Prepare to Kindle Your Inner Fire Again:

At the conclusion of this chapter, you will have the understanding necessary to:

Dispel the fallacy about metabolism and discover the real causes of weight gain.

Determine the true offenders in your personal attempt to lose weight.

Put more effort into enhancing your metabolic health in order to achieve long-term success.

Here's your time to take back authority and cease falling for the "slow metabolism" myth. Together, we can ignite your inner flame and unleash your maximum metabolic potential. Let's get started!

Busting the Belly Bulge: Dispelling Often Held Myths About Metabolism

Have you ever had the impression that all it would take to see the weight gain was one glance at a cupcake? Have you been informed that losing weight is unattainable and that your metabolism is "broken"? Wait a moment! Let us dispel some of the most common misconceptions about metabolism that hold individuals back before they give up and live a life of lettuce leaves and hopelessness.

Myth No. 1: Your Metabolism Is "Slow" for Life Genetics do play a part, but it's not a death sentence! Building muscle mass via strength exercise can actually speed up your metabolism since muscle burns more calories than fat.

Myth No. 2: Your metabolism slows down if you eat after 7 PM. Actually, it depends on what you eat, not when. Pizza binges at midnight will undoubtedly impede your progress, but you may keep your metabolism going and avoid cravings at night by having a nutritious snack before bed.

Myth No. 3: Spicy Foods is a Magic Bullet for Losing Weight Although a little increase in body temperature is possible with chili peppers, it is not a substantial enough increase to be a permanent fix. For long-lasting effects, concentrate on forming healthful behaviors.

Myth No. 4: Not Eating Increases Metabolism Self-starvation is really counterproductive! Your body enters "starvation mode" and will stop at nothing to hold onto calories. For a healthy, well-balanced metabolism, aim for frequent meals.

Myth No. 5: Your Body Is a Detoxing Machine Already! Certain "Detox" Drinks or Supplements Can Fix a Slow Metabolism There's no fast remedy or miracle potion. For the best metabolic health, prioritize a well-balanced diet, consistent exercise, and adequate sleep.

Are You All Set to Bust the Myths and Boost Your Metabolism?

This book will serve as your resource for comprehending your metabolism, dispelling the fallacies that are preventing you from reaching your goals, and developing a long-term, sustainable weight reduction and health strategy. Prepare to let go of fads, adopt a healthy diet, and unleash the potential of your incredible metabolism!

Finding the Causes of Your Weight Gain: Deciphering Your Metabolism's Code

Feeling trapped when trying to lose weight? It appears as though the scale is determined to resist your attempts, leaving you perplexed and angry. However, what if the source of the issue isn't a "broken" metabolism but rather a covert actor operating behind the scenes?

We'll go on a detective hunt to find the underlying reasons for weight gain in this chapter. We'll reveal the unexpected elements that might undermine your good intentions and cause the weight to continue to gain.

Prepare to explore:

The Metabolism Myth: Dispelling the fallacy that people have a "slow metabolism" and exposing the real story behind this amazing mechanism.

The Sneaky Saboteurs: Exposing the covert offenders—such as stress hormones, sleep disorders, and even certain medications—that can thwart your attempts to lose weight.

Diet Deception: Understanding the complex world of food and recognizing dietary practices that promote weight gain, such as portion control issues and hidden sweets.

The Gut Connection: Examining the intriguing relationship between metabolism and gut health as well as the potential impact of your gut microbiota on weight.

Personalized Solutions: Giving you the tools to manage the particular factors that lead to weight gain and unleash the potential for natural fat burning in your body.

This chapter is a revelation rather than merely a collection of facts! You'll get the information and resources necessary to pinpoint the underlying issues that are unique to you, enabling you to design a customized weight-management strategy.

Are you prepared to truly unlock the secrets of your metabolism and lose weight for good? Let's make a change and discover the keys to a happy, healthier self!

Chapter 3: Macronutrients: Your Body's Power house's Building Blocks

Put an end to boring diet terminology and constrictive menus! We'll unlock the mysteries of macronutrients, the extraordinary elements that power your incredible body, in this chapter. We'll show you how these macro heroes combine to help you burn fat, gain muscle, and maintain your energy levels all day.

Let's first discuss the macro- and micronutrients found in diet.

Nutrients in diet are vital elements that sustain growth, facilitate energy production, aid in tissue repair, and control physiological processes. They consist of water, vitamins, minerals, proteins, fats, and carbs.

Macronutrients: These are the main nutrients your body requires in big amounts for energy: carbs, proteins, and fats. Food nutrients is a larger word that includes all the ingredients in food that your body needs to function.

Micronutrients: These include vitamins, minerals, and other elements that are required in much lower amounts but are nevertheless vital for many body processes.

A more precise word, macronutrients, only describes the abundance of nutrients that supply the majority of your body's energy.

Therefore, not all food nutrients are macronutrients, even if all macronutrients are food nutrients.

The Three Magnificent Elements: Fat, Protein, and Carbs

Think of your body as an opulent house. Protein is the steel that makes sturdy buildings, fat is the insulator that keeps everything moving smoothly, and carbs are the bricks that give a firm foundation. Unlocking your maximum potential requires an awareness of the distinct qualities of each macronutrient, which plays a crucial role.

Imagine carbohydrates as the fuel that keeps your engine going. They are your body's main source of energy. Your body effectively transforms them into glucose, which powers your muscles and brain. However, not every carb is made equal! We'll discuss the distinction between simple carbohydrates, which can cause blood sugar spikes and crashes, and complex carbohydrates, which offer steady energy.

Protein is the superhero of the nutritional world. It is a muscle-building marvel. It serves as the foundation for nearly all of your body's tissues, including muscles and bones. Your body converts protein that you ingest into amino acids, which are subsequently needed for tissue growth and repair. We'll get into the many forms of protein sources and how to make sure you're receiving enough to maintain a robust physique and a fast metabolism.

Don't Be Afraid of Fat! - Fat has been blamed as the primary cause of weight gain for many years. However, the fact is that a number of body processes depend on healthy fats. They maintain hormone synthesis, provide you with steady energy, and prolong feelings of fullness. We will discuss the types of fats—good, bad, and healthy—and how to include them in your diet to get the best possible health.

Constructing Your Powerhouse of Macronutrients.

Now that you are aware of the stars, it's time to create your own customized macronutrient strategy! We'll offer a detailed how-to for:
Identifying your specific needs: We'll work with you to ascertain the right proportion of carbohydrates, protein, and fat for your body based on your objectives and degree of activity.

In this lesson, we will teach you how to construct gourmet meals that delight your taste buds and fulfill your macronutrient requirements. We will throw out the boring constraints and show you how to build meals that are both delicious and balanced.
You may get ideas for your meals by looking at a selection of example meal plans that are designed to accommodate a variety of dietary preferences and objectives.
Your Key to a Healthier and More Vibrant You Is Found in the Macronutrient Program
Through a knowledge and mastery of macronutrients, you will be able to access a wealth of advantages, including the following:

Your metabolism may be revved up by maintaining the appropriate balance of macronutrients, which will allow you to burn more calories throughout the day while you are eating.

It's time to say goodbye to yo-yo dieting and achieve sustainable weight management! The basis for weight loss that is both healthy and possible to maintain is provided by macronutrients.

Improved Energy Levels: Say goodbye to exhaustion in the afternoon! You will be able to maintain your strength and energy levels by consuming a balanced combination of macronutrients.

A balanced intake of macronutrients helps general well-being in a number of ways, including the promotion of hormonal equilibrium and the maintenance of healthy muscular tissue.

So, are you ready to abandon the diet confusion and harness the power of macronutrients? Let's go on this exciting adventure together and strengthen your body's powerhouse for a healthier, more vibrant you!

Understanding Macronutrients: Carbs, Protein, and Fat - The Fuel Fight Club for Your Health!

Imagine your body as a high-performance machine. To keep it functioning optimally, you need the correct fuel. That's where macronutrients come in: the carbohydrates, protein, and fat that play a major role in your health and weight control. But these aren't your usual gladiators slugging it out in a nutritious arena. They're a potent trio, each with specific capabilities that, when used intelligently, may unleash enormous health benefits.

In this chapter, we'll enter the interesting realm of macronutrients, decoding their mysteries and refuting the misconceptions. Get ready to:

Unmask the Macronutrient Mafia: We'll disclose the reality behind carbohydrates, protein, and fat, separating fact from myth. Learn why carbohydrates aren't the enemy, why protein isn't just for bodybuilders, and why fat deserves a place on your plate.

Discover Their Superpowers: Each macronutrient brings a distinct set of benefits to the table. We'll look into how carbs feed your energy, protein develops and repairs tissues, while fat keeps you feeling content and supports important activities.

Craft Your Winning Combo: Not all macros are made equal. Depending on your objectives and lifestyle, you'll learn how to design a tailored macronutrient profile that maintains your body performing at its optimum.

Boss Your Meals: Forget restrictive diets! We'll empower you with the information to make educated decisions about the meals you eat. You'll uncover delicious and healthy alternatives high in each macronutrient to construct a diet that's both effective and fun.

Understanding macronutrients isn't just about counting numbers; it's about enabling you to take care of your health and feed your body for a full, active existence. So, skip the trendy diets and discover the possibilities of a balanced macronutrient approach. Let's get started!

Creating a Balanced Macronutrient Profile for Your Needs: Unlock the Magic Ratio for Your Metabolism.

Dieting might feel like a complex game of restriction and deprivation. But what if the secret to unlocking your metabolic potential wasn't about cutting out entire food categories, but rather generating a symphony of nutrients that function together in harmony? Enter the realm of macronutrients - the building components of your food that play a major role in accelerating your metabolism and feeding your body for a healthier, more energetic you.

we'll unlock the code on macronutrients: carbohydrates, protein, and fat. We'll explore:

The Macronutrient Power Trio: Uncover the unique features of each macronutrient and how they affect your metabolism, energy levels, and general health.

The Not-So-Secret Weapon: The Thermic Effect of Food (TEF): Discover how your body burns calories merely by digesting food, and how protein reigns supreme in this metabolic game.

Building Your Personalized Plate: Learn how to understand food labels and identify the macronutrient makeup of different meals. We'll assist you in designing a balanced macronutrient profile specific to your particular requirements and objectives, whether it's weight reduction, muscle growth, or maintaining optimal health.

Beyond the Basics: Macronutrient Hacks for Success: Ditch the boring diet attitude! We'll uncover great recipe ideas and practical advice to ensure your meals are not just healthful but also overflowing with taste.

Get ready to quit the restrictive fad diets and expose a flexible, sustainable approach to eating that feeds your body, boosts your metabolism, and starts you on the way to a healthier, more vibrant self. So, grab your metaphorical chef's hat, because you're about to become the master of your own destiny!

Chapter 4: The Power of Protein: Unleashing Your Inner Fat-Burning Machine

Imagine a hidden weapon in your struggle for a healthier, smaller you. It's not a fad diet or a miraculous drug, but a powerful vitamin lying in plain sight: protein. Forget the tasteless chicken breasts of yesteryear. Today, we'll explore the intriguing world of protein, unlocking its ability to remodel your metabolism and convert your body into a fat-burning inferno.

Protein: The Building Block of a Boosted Metabolism

Think of your body as a marvelous mechanism. Every activity, from growing muscle to digesting food, requires fuel. Protein is the essential building ingredient for this fuel. Unlike carbohydrates and fats, the body consumes a substantial quantity of calories only to digest and absorb protein - a process termed the thermic effect of food (TEF). It's like your body has a tiny metabolic celebration every time you consume protein!

Here's the interesting part: ingesting enough protein can really raise your resting metabolic rate (RMR). This means your body burns more calories even at rest, establishing a calorie deficit - the critical element for lasting weight reduction.

Beyond the Burn: The Satiety Superpower

Protein isn't simply a metabolic miracle; it's also a satiety superstar. Ever been hungry quickly after a carb-heavy meal? Protein keeps you feeling fuller for longer, decreasing cravings and preventing overeating. This is because protein causes the production of hormones like peptide YY (PYY), which convey signals to your brain that you're full.

Imagine saying goodbye to those afternoon snack attacks and welcome to maintained energy levels throughout the day!

Fueling Your Transformation: Protein Powerhouses

Now, let's get practical. Where can you locate these protein powerhouses? This is a veritable gold mine of delicious choices:

Lean meats and poultry: Chicken breast, turkey breast, lean cuts of beef, and fish.

Seafood: Salmon, tuna, shrimp, and oysters, rich with omega-3 fatty acids for significant health advantages.

Eggs: A complete protein source with all the key amino acids needed for muscular growth.

Plant-based proteins: Beans, lentils, tofu, tempeh, and quinoa — great for vegetarians and vegans.

Remember, diversity is crucial! Explore diverse protein sources to keep your taste buds pleased and your body fueled for achievement.

Unleash Your Inner Fat-Burning Machine: Putting it all Together

So, how much protein is enough? The answer varies on your particular needs, but a decent starting point is 0.8 grams of protein per kilogram of body weight. Consult a trained healthcare practitioner to discover the ideal protein consumption for you.

By including protein wisely into your diet, you'll be well on your way to:

Boosting your metabolism and burning more calories at rest.

Feeling fuller for longer, minimizing cravings and overeating.

Building and maintaining muscular mass further promotes a healthy metabolism.

Embrace the power of protein, and see your body change into a fat-burning powerhouse eager to help your weight reduction quest and general well-being. Remember, the path to a better you is a thrilling adventure, and protein is your powerful partner!

Unleash Your Inner Furnace: How Protein Stoked the Fire of Metabolism

Have you ever wished your body burnt calories like a high-performance engine? Well, guess what? It already does, and protein is the secret fuel that keeps that fire burning!

This chapter goes into the intriguing realm of the Thermic Effect of Food (TEF), uncovering the hidden ability protein holds to enhance your metabolism and convert you into a calorie-burning engine.

Imagine this: you enjoy a beautiful dinner, but the labor doesn't stop there. Your body swings into high gear, breaking down that meal and utilizing some of the energy it pulls especially for that very process! That's TEF in action.

But here's the fun part: not all meals are created equal when it comes to TEF. Protein reigns supreme, demanding a far greater energy expenditure for digestion and absorption compared to carbohydrates or fat. It's like placing a premium log on your metabolic fire — it burns hotter and longer!

Get ready to revolutionize your view on eating! This chapter isn't only about protein; it's about learning how your body operates as a wonderful fat-burning mechanism. With the appropriate information and protein as your ally, you can take charge of your metabolism and ignite a permanent transformation towards a healthier, more energetic self!

Chapter 5: Rethinking Carbs: Not All Carbs Are Created Equal - Ditch the Rollercoaster, Embrace Sustainable Energy!

Carbs: Friend or Foe?

For decades, carbohydrates have been vilified as the reason behind weight gain and slow metabolisms. But hang on a minute! Carbs are absolutely required for our bodies to operate correctly. The answer lies in recognizing the many forms of carbohydrates and making wise choices to nourish your body for maximum health and prolonged energy.

The Glycemic Index: The Ride You Didn't Sign Up For

Imagine your blood sugar as a rollercoaster. Simple carbs, such as sugary beverages and white bread, generate quick rises in blood sugar, followed by a crashing low. This "sugar rush" leaves you feeling depleted and needing more carbs, creating a vicious cycle. But there's wonderful news!

Introducing Complex Carbs: Your Steady Energy Source

Complex carbs, such as whole grains, veggies, and legumes, break down slowly, giving a consistent source of energy throughout the day. Think of them as a mild slope on a picturesque trek, not a heart-stopping ascent. These complex carbohydrates are filled with fiber, which keeps you feeling fuller for longer, aids with digestion, and even helps regulate your metabolism!

Unleashing the Power of Fiber: Your Gut's Best Friend

Fiber is a superhero in the realm of carbohydrates! It functions as a prebiotic, nourishing the beneficial bacteria in your stomach, necessary for a healthy digestive system and general well-being. Not only that, but fiber helps with blood sugar regulation, keeping you feeling active and full.

So, How Do You Choose the Right Carbs?

This chapter will provide you with the information and tools to traverse the world of carbohydrates with confidence. You'll learn:

The Glycemic Index Decoded: Understand how different meals impact your blood sugar and pick wisely.

Fiber Powerhouse Foods: Discover the greatest sources of complex carbohydrates and fiber to feed your body and boost your metabolism.

Carb Counting Made Easy: Learn practical ways to add the proper types of carbohydrates into your diet for long-term weight management and sustained energy.

Delicious, Carb-Conscious Meals: Get inspired with delectable and healthy meals incorporating complex carbohydrates that will keep you feeling satiated and stimulated!

This chapter is not just about carbohydrates — it's about taking control of your energy levels, reaching maximum health, and rejecting the sugar rollercoaster for a path of continuous well-being!

Unveiling the Glycemic Index: Your Cheat Sheet to Blood Sugar Harmony!

Tired of energy crashes? Fed up with feeling lethargic after a meal? Ready to uncover the secrets of stable blood sugar? Then strap up, because we're entering into the intriguing realm of the Glycemic Index (GI)!

This powerful tool will become your secret weapon in regulating your blood sugar and feeding your body for top performance.

Here's what you'll discover:

The Glycemic Index Explained: We'll explain the science underlying the GI, making it simple and easy to grasp. No more uncertainty about weird numbers!

The Food Rollercoaster: Learn how different foods affect your blood sugar levels and how the GI helps you pick intelligently. Say goodbye to energy dips and hello to consistent energy!

Beyond the Basics: Explore the many forms of carbs and their influence on your body. Uncover the hidden sugars lurking in ordinary meals.

Unlock Your Power: Discover how to harness the GI to build a tailored meal plan that keeps your blood sugar regulated and your energy rising.

Delicious Recipes: Forget boring diets! We'll supply you with scrumptious dishes that are both GI-friendly and overflowing with flavor. Eat smart and enjoy the adventure!

This isn't just another dull nutrition lecture. This is a game-changer! Prepare to:

Boost your energy levels and stay energized throughout the day.

Improve your attention and concentration for top mental performance.

Manage your weight easily by making wise eating choices.

Reduce cravings and feel content with healthy, tasty meals.

Promote overall well-being by keeping your blood sugar in balance.

The Glycemic Index: Your Cheat Sheet to Blood Sugar Harmony! Get ready to change your health and uncover a world of vivid vitality and sustained well-being!

Power Up for the Long Haul: Selecting Complex Carbohydrates for Sustained Energy

Forget the midday slump! Dive into the realm of complex carbs, the unsung heroes of prolonged energy. This is your guide to unlocking a consistent source of nourishment for your body and mind.

Here's what you'll discover:

The Crash Course on carbohydrates: We'll break down the difference between basic and complex carbohydrates, explaining why complex choices are your key to enduring energy.

The Glycemic Index: Your Cheat Sheet to Smart Carbs: Learn how this useful tool may help you pick carbs that won't put your blood sugar on a roller coaster trip.

Beyond Bread: A Rainbow of Energy-Boosting Options: Forget the white bread! We'll discover a lively world of tasty and healthful complex carbohydrates, from ancient grains to colorful veggies.

Fueling Your Day: Sample Meal Plans for Peak Performance: Put your newfound knowledge into action with sample meal plans designed to keep you energetic throughout the day.

Unlocking Your Body's Potential: Understand how complex carbohydrates may not only fuel your activities but also boost your general health and well-being.

Get ready to skip the energy drinks and sugar highs! This chapter is your ticket to a world of prolonged energy, greater attention, and a powerful, healthy self.

Chapter 6: Fats: Essential Partners in Metabolism and Overall Health

For years, fat has been stigmatized as the reason behind weight gain and health concerns. But hold the avocado toast! It's time to burst this misconception and disclose the truth: fat is not the enemy — it's a critical ally in your road to a healthier, more vibrant self.

In this chapter, we'll throw light on the intriguing world of fats, exploring:

The Good, the Bad, and the Delicious: Not all fats are made equal. We'll dig into the numerous sorts of fats, from the artery-clogging villains to the metabolism-boosting heroes. Learn how to identify healthy fats you should embrace and bad fats you should politely refuse.

Fat Power: Discover the amazing ways fat nourishes your body. We'll study how fat keeps you feeling fuller for longer, offers continuous energy, and even plays a critical role in brain health and hormone balance.

Fat for a Fit Life: Contrary to common thought, integrating healthy fats into your diet can actually benefit weight management. We'll discuss how fat may boost the thermic effect of food (TEF), thus converting your body into a more efficient calorie-burning machine.

Fat Fighters: Unleash the fat-fighting potential of healthy fats! We'll investigate how certain fats can help reduce inflammation, enhance blood sugar regulation, and even minimize your risk of chronic illnesses.

The Fat Feast: Ready to put your newfound knowledge into action? We'll present a delightful guide to introducing healthy fats into your meals. Discover a world of delectable alternatives that are both beneficial for you and fantastic for your taste buds!

Visualize the different types of fats and their influence on your body.

Debunking myths: We'll clear up common misunderstandings about fat and lay the record straight.

Real-life examples: See how consuming healthy fats may alter your health narrative.

Delicious meals: Get inspired with easy-to-follow recipes displaying the power of healthy fats in action.

Get ready to discard the fear and embrace the fat! By the end of this chapter, you'll be armed with the information and skills to make educated decisions regarding fat, access its health advantages, and experience a new level of energy.

Demystifying the World of Fat: Friends, Foes, and Fuel for Your Body

Fat. It's a term frequently said with a grimace, conjuring thoughts of greasy fast food and expanding waistlines. But hang on a minute! Not all fats are created equal. In reality, some fats are superstars when it comes to your health and weight control.

Get ready to discard the preconceptions and plunge into the intriguing realm of fats! In this chapter, we'll explore the mysteries of these critical nutrients, investigating the many kinds and their unexpected functions in keeping you energized, healthy, and feeling your best.

The Good, the Bad, and the Misunderstood:

First, let's clear the air. We may categorize fats into three primary groups:

The All-Stars: Unsaturated Fats - These are the nice ones! They occur in two forms:

Monounsaturated Fats (MUFAs): Picture the heart-healthy fats in olive oil and avocados. MUFAs can help decrease your "bad" LDL cholesterol while raising your "good" HDL cholesterol, keeping your heart happy.

Polyunsaturated Fats (PUFAs): These champions come in two sub-categories: omega-3 and omega-6 fatty acids. Think of omega-3s as brain enhancers found in fatty seafood like salmon, enhancing memory and lowering inflammation. Omega-6s, abundant in sunflower seeds and vegetable oils, work hand-in-hand with omega-3s for general health.

The Stealthy Villain: Trans Fats: These are the ones to avoid at all costs. Artificially generated during food processing, trans fats elevate bad cholesterol and increase your risk of heart disease. Be on the alert for "partially hydrogenated oils" on food labels — that's a warning signal for trans fats!

The misunderstood One: Saturated Fats: Saturated fats receive a poor name, but they're not all bad news. Found in meat, dairy products, and coconut oil, saturated fats should be eaten in moderation. While they can elevate LDL cholesterol, some sources, like coconut oil, also offer potential health advantages.

Fat Power! How These Essential Nutrients Fuel Your Body:

Now that you know the players, let's discover the fantastic things fats do for you:

Energy Source: Fats are a concentrated source of energy, giving more than twice the calories per gram compared to carbohydrates and protein. This makes them great for sustained energy levels throughout the day.

developing Blocks: Fat serves a critical function in developing and maintaining healthy cells.

Vitamin Absorption: Some vitamins, including A, D, E, and K, are soluble in fat. This implies they need fat for efficient absorption in their body.

Organ Protection: Fat acts as a cushion around your organs, offering crucial protection.

Hormone generation: Fats are important for the generation of hormones that govern many body activities.

Making Smart Fat Choices:

Understanding the different types of fats allows you to make educated decisions about what you put on your plate. Here are some tips:

Focus on Unsaturated Fats: Include lots of MUFAs and PUFAs in your diet from healthy sources including nuts, seeds, olive oil, and fatty seafood.

Limit Saturated Fats: Enjoy them in moderation, preferring lean protein sources and opting for full-fat dairy items less frequently.

Beware of Trans Fats: Read food labels carefully and avoid goods containing partly hydrogenated oils.

Embrace a Balanced Diet: Remember, a healthy diet is all about variety and moderation. Include healthy fats with fruits, veggies, complete grains, and lean protein sources.

By knowing the many types of fats and their responsibilities, you may improve your connection with this crucial nutrient. Embrace the healthy fats, keep the bad ones away, and uncover a world of vigor and well-being!

Unleash Your Inner Fat Burner: Delicious Sources of Healthy Fats to Supercharge Your Metabolism!

For years, fat has been stigmatized as the enemy of weight reduction. But the reality is, that fat is an important macronutrient your body requires for maximum health and a revved-up metabolism!

In this chapter, we'll discover the secrets of good fats, converting them from villain to superhero in your weight reduction quest. Get ready to explore a treasure trove of tasty selections that will:

Boost your metabolism: Certain fats really help your body burn more calories throughout the day! Say welcome to a natural fat-burning edge.

Keep you feeling satisfied: Healthy fats have a staying power, keeping you fuller for longer and eliminating those bothersome cravings that derail your diet.

Support general health: These powerful fats are filled with important elements that contribute to heart health, cognitive function, and hormone balance.

So, shed the fear and delve into this delectable world of good-for-you fats!

The All-Star Lineup: Your Healthy Fat Shopping List

The Mighty Monounsaturated Fats: These superstars like avocados, olive oil, and nuts give a one-two punch - increasing metabolism and keeping you feeling satiated. Guacamole, anyone? Drizzle some olive oil on your veggies, or have a handful of nuts for a heart-healthy snack.

The Omega-3 Powerhouse: Fatty fish like salmon, mackerel, and sardines are champions for a reason! Packed with omega-3 fatty acids, they prevent inflammation, enhance cognitive function, and even help in fat burning. Two servings a week may make a lot of difference.

The Seed Sensation: Chia seeds, flaxseeds, and pumpkin seeds are little nutritional powerhouses filled with healthy fats, fiber, and protein. Sprinkle them over your yogurt, or porridge, or even bake them into muffins for a pleasant and nutritious crunch.

Don't Forget the Dairy Delights: Full-fat yogurt and cheese (select low-sodium varieties) are fantastic providers of healthful fats, calcium, and protein. Enjoy a dab of Greek yogurt with berries for breakfast, or add cheese to a balanced salad for a delicious lunch.

Remember: Moderation is crucial! While these fats are wonderful, having them as part of a balanced diet is vital.

Get Creative in the Kitchen: Experiment with these healthy fats to make tasty and fulfilling meals. Roast veggies with olive oil and herbs, throw up a smoothie with avocado and nut butter or indulge in some baked fish with a lemon-dill sauce.

Embrace the Power of Fat! By including these healthy fat sources into your diet, you'll not only be pleasing your taste senses but also feeding your body for maximum health and a naturally increased metabolism. So, release your inner fat burner and go on a tasty road to a healthier, happier self!

Chapter 7: Cracking the Calorie Code: Unlock Sustainable Weight Loss

Imagine a world where weight reduction seems less like a war and more like a victory lap. In this chapter, we'll disclose the hidden weapon in your weight reduction arsenal: the calorie deficit. But forget crash diets and excessive calorie restriction. Here, we'll crack the calorie code, teaching you how to develop a sustainable plan that nourishes your body and burns fat for good.

The Calorie Balancing Act:

Our bodies are like perfectly tuned engines. Calories operate as the fuel, propelling our every motion and thought. The secret to weight loss rests in recognizing this equilibrium. Our bodies retain extra calories as fat when we consume more than we burn off. Conversely, a calorie deficit — burning more calories than we consume – leads to our body tapping into stored fat for energy, resulting in weight loss.

But It's Not Just About Numbers:

Sure, tracking calories may be a beneficial tool. But it's not the complete tale. We'll investigate the topic of calorie quality. Not all calories are created equal! A bag of chips could contain the same number of calories as a grilled chicken breast, but their impact on your body is dramatically different. We'll go into the realm of macronutrients — protein, carbohydrates, and fat – and how to build a balanced plate that keeps you feeling pleased and energized while supporting your weight reduction objectives.

Finding Your Calorie Sweet Spot:

This chapter won't be a one-size-fits-all approach. We'll take you through determining your Basal Metabolic Rate (BMR) - the number of calories your body burns at rest – and then add in your activity level to establish your daily calorie needs. But don't worry, we won't leave you with incomprehensible formulae! We'll give easy-to-use charts, calculators, and examples to help you locate your personal calorie sweet spot.

Making Calorie Deficits Work for You:

Creating a lasting calorie deficit isn't about deprivation. It's about wise decisions and portion management. We'll teach practical techniques to make healthy choices, avoid hidden calorie hazards, and handle social settings without derailing your success.

This Chapter Will Help You:

Understand the notion of calorie balance and its function in weight loss.

Learn how to determine your daily calorie needs.

Discover the relevance of macronutrients and make smart dietary choices.

Develop healthy behaviors and portion management tactics for lasting weight loss.

Feel empowered to develop a tailored calorie deficit strategy that matches your lifestyle.

Recall that losing weight is a journey rather than a goal. By unlocking the calorie code, you'll unlock the secret to long-term success. Let's forsake the fad diets and stringent measures. In this chapter, we'll equip you with the information and techniques to build a sustained calorie deficit that nourishes your body and keeps you energetic on the way to a healthier, happier self!

Demystifying the Magic Number: Understanding Calories and Daily Needs

Unleash Your Body's Inner Powerhouse!

Have you ever felt lost in a sea of calorie labels and contradicting dietary advice? Do you wonder what that figure on the nutrition information panel actually signifies for your weight loss quest or general health? Fear not! This chapter is the key to uncovering the secrets of calories and daily demands. Get ready to:

Bust the Calorie Myth: We'll refute the misunderstanding of calories as just "energy units" and investigate their deeper influence on your metabolism.

Fuel Your Machine: Discover how your body uses calories for diverse activities, from fueling your brain to producing powerful muscles.

The Personalized Equation: Learn how factors like age, exercise level, and even heredity impact your daily calorie needs.

No More Calorie Counting Drudgery: We'll examine alternate ways for mindful eating and portion control, making healthy choices a breeze.

Unlock Your Metabolic Potential: Dive into how your everyday activities and dietary choices may impact your metabolic rate, the key to burning more calories at rest.

Get ready for interactive components!

Calorie Calculator Challenge: Take a fun quiz to estimate your own daily calorie needs depending on your lifestyle.

Food Detective Game: Analyze food labels together, determining calorie content and making smart decisions.

The "Fuel Gauge" Experiment: Track your energy levels throughout the day and discover how they connect with your calorie consumption.

This chapter will not only arm you with information but also empower you to take command of your gasoline tank. By knowing calories and daily demands, you'll be well on your way to:

Achieving Optimal Weight Management: Learn how to generate a sustainable calorie deficit for healthy and permanent weight reduction.

Fueling Peak Performance: Discover the correct calorie balance to enhance your energy levels throughout the day.

Optimizing Your Health: Understand how a balanced calorie intake leads to general well-being and illness prevention.

So fasten your seatbelts and get ready for an exciting voyage! We're about to alter the way you perceive calories - from confused numbers to powerful tools for a healthier, more vibrant you!

Crack the Calorie Code: Develop Your Personalized Fat-Burning Blueprint!

Tired of basic diet regimens that leave you disappointed and hungry?

Unlock the key to sustained weight reduction and long-term health with a tailored calorie control strategy developed just for YOU! This chapter is your key to:

Understanding your body's specific needs: Learn how factors like age, exercise level, and body composition impact your calorie requirements.

Ditching the calorie guessing game: Discover a step-by-step technique to calculate your precise daily calorie budget for weight reduction, maintenance, or muscle building.

Fueling your body for success: Explore the science behind macronutrients (carbs, protein, fat) and how to construct a tailored macro diet that optimizes metabolism and keeps you feeling energized.

Building flexibility: Learn ways to adjust your diet based on activity levels, travel, and social engagements - no more strict meal plans!

Beyond the numbers: Explore the psychological components of mindful eating to create a healthy relationship with food and avoid cravings.

Get ready to:

Unleash your body's fat-burning potential!

Experience continuous energy throughout the day!

Say goodbye to yo-yo dieting and welcome to a healthier, happier you!

This chapter is packed with interesting activities, insightful infographics, and real-life examples to help you adapt your calorie control strategy for success. You'll also uncover great meal ideas that meet your individual macros, making healthy eating a breeze.

Are you ready to crack the calorie code and unlock your full potential? Let's plunge in!

Chapter 8: Exercise for Metabolic Enhancement: Moving Your Body for Long-Term Benefits

Forget the trendy exercises and crash diets! Unleash your body's inherent fat-burning furnace with the power of movement. In this chapter, we'll dig into the exciting realm of exercise for metabolic optimization, teaching you how to unleash a healthier, more energetic self.

From Couch Potato to Calorie-Crushing Machine:

Imagine this: every stride you take, every push-up you achieve, becomes a weapon in your armor against slow metabolism.Exercise isn't only about looks;

it's a metabolic transformation! We'll explore:

The Science Behind the Sweat: Discover how different forms of exercise – from heart-pumping aerobic to muscle-building strength training – convert your body into a calorie-burning engine. Learn about EPOC (Excess Post-exercise Oxygen Consumption) — the afterburn effect that keeps your metabolism going even after you've stopped moving.

Building a Muscle Machine: Muscle is metabolically costly tissue. Your body burns more calories at rest if it is more muscular! We'll break down the finest strength training routines to shape a lean body and enhance your metabolism.

exercise: Your Fat-Burning Engine: Get your heart racing with intense exercise programs that will blaze calories and leave you feeling refreshed. We'll teach you how to locate workouts you genuinely love so that working out becomes fun, not a job.

Beyond the Gym: Unleash Your Inner Athlete Everywhere!

Exercise doesn't have to be restricted to the gym walls. This chapter will open a treasure trove of imaginative methods to get your body moving and your metabolism revving:

Turn Your Commute into a Calorie Burner: Swap the automobile for a bike ride or a brisk walk. You'll save money, decrease stress, and enhance your metabolism — triple win!

Take the Stairs, Challenge Yourself: Forget the elevator! Opting for the stairs is a simple yet efficient strategy to include bursts of action throughout your day.

Deskercise Revolution: Sitting all day may wreak havoc on your metabolism. We'll teach you basic desk workouts to keep your body active during the workday.

Make Exercise a Habit for Life:

This chapter is about developing a sustainable fitness regimen that you can keep to. We'll provide you with tips on:

Finding Your Fitness Fun: Find things that you truly like, such as dancing, swimming, or hiking. Exercise should not feel like a punishment!

Setting Realistic Goals: Don't expect to transform from couch potato to marathon runner overnight. Set attainable objectives and celebrate your accomplishments along the way.

Creating a Support System: Find a workout partner or attend a fitness class. Having someone to encourage you may make a huge impact.

Get ready to experience:

Higher energy levels

improved sleep quality.

Stronger muscles and bones

You'll feel more confident and empowered!

Exercise is more than just burning calories; it is a long-term investment in your health and well-being. So, lace up your shoes, turn on your favorite soundtrack, and prepare to unleash the wonderful power of movement!

Unleash Your Inner Hercules: Strength Training and Muscle Mass

Tired of feeling scrawny? Are you ready to reject the "skinny jeans" moniker for good?

This book isn't only about growing muscle; it's about realizing your entire potential. It is about altering your body and mind via the force of strength training. Forget endless aerobics and trendy diets; strength training is the secret to being stronger, healthier, and more confident.

Here's what you'll find inside.

The Science of Strength: Delve into the intriguing topic of muscle growth and discover how to optimize your body's capacity to generate lean muscle mass.

The Ultimate Muscle-Building Blueprint: Forget basic training routines! Create a personalized strength training program based on your objectives and fitness level.

Unlocking Hidden Power: To keep your workouts difficult and fun, try a range of training approaches, including bodyweight exercises, free weights, and machines.

Fueling Your Fire: Learn about dietary techniques that are particularly intended to promote muscular growth and recovery. Avoid restrictive diets and learn how to eat for results.

Beyond the Iron: Discover the psychological advantages of strength training. Experience more confidence, a better mood, and a warrior attitude.

Smashing Through Plateaus: Discover how to detect and conquer plateaus, keeping your muscle-building progress on track.

Real-World Examples: Be inspired by the success stories of people who have altered their lives with strength training.

This book provides a comprehensive guide to developing a strong, healthy physique. It includes instructive pictures, simple explanations, and practical recommendations to help you reach your fitness objectives and release your inner Hercules (or Hera!).

Are you ready to begin a journey of strength and transformation? Let's get started.

Get Pumped, Get Fired Up: How Cardio Boosts Metabolism for Weight Loss and Wellness!

Tired of feeling sluggish? Want to make your body a calorie-burning machine? Look no further than the benefits of cardiac exercise! This thrilling chapter delves deeply into the realm of cardio, exposing its secrets for increasing your metabolism and unlocking a healthier, more energetic self.

Here's what you'll uncover.

The Metabolic Afterburn Effect: Unleash the secret magic of exercise that keeps your body burning calories long after you finish working out! We'll explain the science behind this fat-burning phenomenon.

Don't worry if you're a beginner at exercising! We'll look at a variety of aerobic activities suitable for all fitness levels, including brisk walking, swimming, dancing, and group fitness programs.

Unlock Your Inner Athlete: Experience the thrill of movement! Learn how to identify activities you enjoy, break through fitness plateaus, and remain motivated for long-term success.

Beyond Weight Loss: The Incredible Health Benefits of Exercise: We'll look beyond the scale to see how exercise strengthens your heart, improves your mood, increases your energy levels, and even fights disease.

The Personalized Cardio Plan: This is not a one-size-fits-all strategy! We'll help you design a personalized cardio plan that works around your schedule, preferences, and fitness objectives.

Get ready for:

Feel the difference as cardio pushes oxygen throughout your body, leaving you energized and ready to tackle the day.

Blast stubborn fat: Learn how exercise may help you burn stored fat and build lean muscle, resulting in a more contoured and healthy physique.

Sleep like a champ: Regular exercise encourages deeper, more restful sleep, leaving you feeling energized and ready to tackle the day.

Sharpen your mind: Prepare for a cognitive boost! Cardio increases blood flow to the brain, which enhances attention, memory, and general cognitive performance.

Invest in your future: Discover how regular cardio can lower your chance of chronic illnesses such as heart disease, diabetes, and even some malignancies.

This chapter will help you become a healthier and happier version of yourself! So put on your sneakers, lace up your enthusiasm, and prepare to discover the transformational power of cardiovascular exercise.

Chapter 9: Sleep and Stress Management: Key Elements for Optimal Metabolism

Unlock the Power of how Sleep and Stress Can Boost Your Metabolism,

Have you ever wondered why, despite eating all the proper meals and exercising diligently, the weight stubbornly remains on? The answer may surprise you. It's not only about consuming and expending calories; it's about building an environment within your body that burns fat effectively. Enter the dynamic combo of sleep and stress management. These often-overlooked elements play an important part in controlling your metabolism, and adjusting them might be the key to maximizing your body's fat-burning capabilities.

Sleep is your body's metabolic recharge station. Imagine your body is a high-performance machine. To perform properly, it needs frequent rest and maintenance, just like any other equipment. This is when sleep comes in.

Your body isn't just sleeping; it's going through a symphony of metabolic activities. Here's how a good night's sleep boosts your metabolism:

Hormonal Harmony: Sleep controls hormone synthesis, including leptin (which promotes fullness) and ghrelin (which stimulates appetite). When you don't get enough sleep, your ghrelin levels rise, making you want unhealthy meals and making it difficult to feel satisfied.

Muscle Building and Repair: As you sleep, your body produces growth hormone, which is essential for muscle tissue development and repair. Muscle is metabolically active, which means it burns more calories even while resting.

Prioritize sleep to become a slim, calorie-burning machine!

Cellular Optimization: Deep sleep permits your body to eliminate cellular waste, which can hamper metabolic activity. Consider it a spring cleaning for your cells, ensuring that they operate smoothly and effectively.

Stress: The Metabolism Wrecker and How to Manage It

Chronic stress is the antithesis of a healthy metabolism. When stressed, your body produces cortisol, a hormone that activates the "fight-or-flight" response. This survival mechanism redirects energy away from digestion and metabolism to prepare you for a perceived attack. Here's the issue: in today's society, stress frequently becomes chronic, resulting in

Elevated Cortisol Levels: Chronic cortisol causes your body to constantly "burn sugar for energy," which can lead to blood sugar abnormalities and weight gain.

Increased desires: Stress can cause desires for sweet and fatty meals, making it difficult to make healthy choices.

Disrupted Sleep: Stress can make it harder to fall and remain asleep, resulting in a vicious cycle that disturbs your metabolism.

Relaxation and Its Metabolic Benefits

The good news: you have the ability to regulate stress and get its metabolic advantages. Here are some effective relaxing techniques:

Deep Breathing Exercises: Simple yet effective. Deep, calm breaths trigger your body's relaxation response, which reduces cortisol levels and promotes better sleep.

Mindfulness and meditation: Focusing on the present moment helps to relax the mind and lower stress hormones. There are several mindfulness applications and guided meditations accessible online.

Regular Exercise: Physical activity is an excellent stress reducer. Even modest activity, such as brisk walking, can considerably lower cortisol levels.

Prioritize Sleep Hygiene: Create a pleasant nighttime ritual to guarantee restful sleep. Set a consistent sleep routine, establish a relaxing sleep environment, and avoid using devices before bed.

Conclusion: Sleep well, de-stress, and ignite your metabolism.

Prioritizing sleep and adopting stress management practices into your daily routine not only benefits your health but also builds a metabolic powerhouse. With more sleep and less stress, your hormones will be in balance, your cravings will be under control, and your body will be poised for effective calorie burning. So, switch off the devices, take a deep breath, and prepare to feel the transforming effects of sleep and stress management on your metabolism and general health!

Unleash Your Inner Fat-Burning Machine with the Secret Weapon of Sleep

Ever wonder why that extra slice of cake lingers on your hips after a long night? It is not just your imagination! Quality sleep is the quiet custodian of your metabolism, the key to unlocking your body's inherent fat-burning powerhouse. But how does sleep do its magic? Buckle up, because we're about to delve into the intriguing science of sleep and its remarkable effect on metabolic health.

Sleep: The Metabolic Mastermind.

While you drift off to dreamland, your body is not idle. It's in the process of profound regeneration, fine-tuning a complex symphony of hormones that control how your body utilizes energy. Here's how sleep fires up your metabolism:

The Insulin Advantage: During deep sleep, your body produces more insulin, the hormone that transports glucose (sugar) from your bloodstream to your cells, where it is utilized for energy. This leads to better blood sugar management and a lower chance of insulin resistance, which plays a crucial role in weight growth and type 2 diabetes.

The development of Hormone Boost: This wonder hormone is created during sleep and supports muscle development and repair. Muscle tissue burns more calories at rest, acting as your body's natural fat-burning furnace. So, the more quality sleep you receive, the more muscle you gain, and the faster your metabolism!

The Leptin/Ghrelin Tango: These two hormones control appetite and satiety. When you're sleep deprived, your body generates less leptin (the "I'm full" signal) and more ghrelin (the "I'm hungry" signal), causing you to seek unhealthy meals and maybe overeat.

Sleep deprivation: The Metabolic Mayhem Maker

If you don't get enough sleep, your metabolic party will become a chaotic disaster. What happens when you don't prioritize sleep?

Stress Hormone Havoc: Sleep deprivation causes an increase in cortisol, the stress hormone. Cortisol encourages fat accumulation, particularly around the stomach, and can even cause increased appetites for sweet and fatty meals.

Metabolic Slowdown: When you are sleep-deprived, your body enters half-conservation mode, slowing your metabolism to preserve energy. This means you'll burn fewer calories throughout the day, making it more difficult to reduce or maintain a healthy weight.

The power is in your hands (and pillow!)

Are you ready to release your inner fat-burning machine? Here's the good news: you have the ability to improve your sleep and get the wonderful metabolic advantages it provides!

Aim for 7-8 hours: Most individuals require 7-8 hours of decent sleep each night. Prioritize a consistent sleep pattern, including on weekends, to help your body manage its normal sleep-wake cycles.

Make your bedroom a sleep sanctuary. Keep it dark, quiet, cool, and clutter-free. Purchase a comfortable pillow and mattress.

Power Down Before Bedtime: Avoid using displays (phones, computers, and televisions) for at least an hour before bedtime. Blue light can interfere with the generation of melatonin, a hormone required for sleep.

Relaxation Rituals: Create a nightly routine that includes taking a warm bath, reading a book, or doing easy stretches. Your body will take this as a cue to relax.

Prioritizing excellent sleep not only provides your body with the rest it requires but also boosts your metabolism, putting you on track to a healthier, happier you! So turn out the lights, harness the magic of sleep, and watch your body change into a sleek, mean fat-burning machine!

De-Stress for Success: Overcome Chaos and Unleash Your Inner Calm

Feeling overwhelmed? Drowning in deadlines and everyday drama? It's time to take back control!

This chapter reveals a wealth of effective stress-reduction tactics and methods for cultivating inner calm. No more white-knuckling your way through life. Imagine:

Improved attention and laser-like productivity

Improved sleep, leaving you feeling refreshed and ready to face anything.

Increased emotional resilience, and easier recovery from adversity.

Improved relationships, promoting greater bonds with loved ones.

This is more than just feeling better; it's about reaching your full potential and thriving in all aspects of life. So, eliminate the stress monster and embrace the following practical strategies:

1. Become a Body Whisperer and Master the Mind-Body Connection.

Deep Breathing Decoded: Use the power of your breath to trigger your body's relaxation reaction. Learn basic breathing techniques to relieve tension in minutes.

Progressive Muscle Relaxation: Imagine the stress leaving your body one muscle group at a time. Discover this specific strategy for relieving physical stress and calming your nervous system.

The Magic of Mindfulness: Discover how to quiet your mind and become present in the moment. Mindfulness methods such as meditation can help to reduce stress and increase concentration.

2. Move It or Lose Stress:

Exercise: Your Body's Natural Stress Relief: Engage in enjoyable activities to get your heart rate up and endorphins flowing. Find the exercise that makes you happy and relieves tension, whether it's dancing or going trekking.

Yoga is an ancient practice that blends physical postures, breathing exercises, and meditation to provide a holistic approach to stress management.

3. Fuel Your Calm: The Food-Mood Connection.

Avoid Stress-Inducing Snacks: Sugar crashes and processed meals can worsen anxiety. Discover good eating habits to fuel your body and mind for maximum stress resilience.

Hydration is critical: dehydration can exacerbate stress symptoms. Learn how to remain hydrated throughout the day for the best health.

4. Laughter is the best medicine.

The Power of Play: Engage in enjoyable activities to lighten and raise your mood. Laughter therapy is a genuine thing, so locate comedy in your daily life and watch the tension melt away.

Spend Time with Loved Ones: Social connection is essential for emotional health. Increase your support network and connect with people that make you laugh and feel valued.

5. Declutter Your Mind and Space:

Tame the To-Do List: Do you feel overwhelmed by your tasks? Learn how to prioritize and develop manageable action plans so you can conquer your day without feeling overwhelmed.

Organize Your Oasis: A messy environment can increase stress. Declutter your living area to create a relaxing refuge.

Remember that stress management is a skill that requires practice, just like any other. Incorporating these tactics into your daily routine can help you become a calmer, more resilient person, ready to face life's problems with grace and confidence.

Chapter 10: Hydration: Unleash Your Inner Powerhouse!

Have you ever felt sluggish, foggy-brained, or like you're dragging through the day? It might not be a shortage of coffee, but rather a quiet enemy: dehydration. Forget the six-pack abs; proper hydration is the hidden weapon for achieving your body's maximum potential!

This chapter is about more than just drinking water (although that is vital). We'll delve deeply into the intriguing topic of hydration, discovering:

The H2Oh-So-Important Role of Water: Learn how water is the lifeblood of every cell in your body, affecting everything from brain function to digestion. Discover why dehydration can cause signs of aging and weariness.

Beyond Water: The Electrolyte Advantage: We'll look at the dynamic pair of water and electrolytes, and how they work together to keep your body working efficiently. Discover how electrolytes energize your muscles, manage your neurological system, and even affect your mood!

The Myth Busters: Dehydration Debunked: We'll dispel popular myths regarding hydration. Learn why thirst alone isn't the greatest signal, and how factors such as activity, weather, and even drugs can affect your water requirements.

Hydration Hacks for the Busy Bee: Life is hectic, but being hydrated does not have to be difficult! We'll give you a toolbox full of practical ideas and tactics for making water your go-to beverage, including flavoring hacks and hydration reminders.

Hydrate Like a Pro: Tracking Your Success: Discover how to tailor your hydration strategy and track your success. Discover entertaining and practical ways to monitor your water consumption and celebrate your accomplishments!

Are you ready to reach your body's maximum potential? Let us transform you into a well-oiled machine, one delicious drink at a time! This Chapter will be your ultimate guide to unlocking the power of hydration, leaving you feeling energetic, focused, and ready to face your day!

The Power of Water: Fueling Your Body's Internal Furnace

Water. It's the very core of life, quenching our thirst and keeping us cool on a hot day. But did you know water plays a starring role in a secret story happening inside you every single second: the amazing process of metabolism?

Think of your body as a boiler, constantly burning fuel (food) to produce energy. Water is the important factor that keeps this furnace operating at its peak. In this chapter, we'll dive deep into the interesting world of water and metabolism, discovering the secrets to unlocking a faster burn and a healthier you.

Water: The Universal Solvent

Imagine a busy marketplace where millions of tiny deals occur every second. This marketplace is the inside of your cell, and water is the busy seller. Water works as a global solvent, dissolving important nutrients from your food, like vitamins, minerals, and glucose, and transporting them throughout your body. Without this efficient transport system, your cells would be starved of the building blocks they need to work properly, leading to sluggish metabolism and lowered energy levels.

The Metabolic Boost: Hydrolysis Takes the Stage

Now, let's get down to the real action - the breakdown of food into useful energy. This process, called hydrolysis, relies heavily on water. Think of it as a magic trick. Water works as a magician's helper, splitting complicated food molecules like carbohydrates and proteins into smaller, simpler ones that your body can easily take and use for fuel. Without enough water, this metabolic magic trick falters, leaving you feeling tired and hurting your weight loss goals.

Flushing Out the Toxins: Water, the Body's Cleanser

Your body is constantly working to remove waste products created during metabolism.

Water plays a key role in this cleansing process. Imagine your body as a city. Water acts as the cleaning system, flushing out toxins and waste products through sweat and pee. When you're dehydrated, this waste removal system becomes clogged, leading to a buildup of toxins that can slow down digestion and impact your general health.

Hydration: The Key to Unlocking Your Metabolic Potential

So, how much water do you need to keep your digestive fire burning bright? The answer varies on several things, but a good rule of thumb is to drink eight glasses of water per day. However, pay attention to your body's cues! Feeling thirsty or feeling tiredness can be signs of dehydration. Amp up your water intake during activity and on hot days to replace lost fluids.

Beyond Water: Hydration Hacks for the Busy Lifestyles

We all lead busy lives, and sometimes, remembering to drink enough water can fall by the wayside. The following advice can help you keep hydrated all day long:

Infuse your water: Add pieces of lemon, cucumber, or berries for a refreshing change.

Carry a reusable water bottle: Keep it by your side as a steady reminder to sip.

Download a drinking app: These apps can track your water intake and send you reminders to drink.

Make water your go-to beverage: Ditch sugary drinks and choose water instead.

The Final Sip: Unlocking a Vibrant You

By choosing water and keeping hydrated, you're not just quenching your thirst, you're feeding your body's internal furnace. Water improves food delivery, boosts metabolism, and flushes out toxins, leading to improved energy levels, a sharper mind, and a healthier you. So, raise a glass to water - the hidden star of your metabolic journey!

Conquer Your Day: Unleash the Power of Hydration!

Tired of feeling sluggish? Drained of energy by afternoon? Your body might be giving you a secret message – it's thirsty!

Water isn't just some boring beverage; it's the lifeblood of your entire system. Unlock your body's secret potential by learning the art of staying hydrated throughout the day.

This guide will be your personal water hero, packed with:

The Shocking Truth About Hydration: Discover how dehydration quietly sabotages your energy, brainpower, and even your workouts!

The H2-Oh-Yeah! Hacks: Learn clever tips and tricks to make water your go-to drink and ditch sugary traps. Infuse your water with delicious flavors, make a personalized hydration plan, and turn water breaks into energizing mini-rituals.

Become a Hydration Mastermind: Unravel the science behind hydration, understand how your body uses water, and spot the sneaky signs that you're thirsty (it's not just thirst!).

Boost Your Health From the Inside Out: Dive into the amazing benefits of optimal hydration – from glowing skin and better focus to improved digestion and weight management.

Hydration for Champions: Level up your workouts! Learn how proper hydration boosts your exercise goals and helps you heal faster.

This isn't just about drinking water; it's about opening a whole new level of you!

Are you ready to ditch the tiredness, unlock your energy stores, and feel the power of optimal hydration? Let's raise a glass (of water, of course!) to a healthier, happier, and more energetic you!

Chapter 11: Fuel Your Fire: Sample Meal Plans for Every Body!

Ready to ditch the one-size-fits-all diet and unlock a world of delicious, metabolism-boosting meals suited to YOU? Buckle up! This chapter is your individual path to success, packed with exciting sample meal plans that cater to various dietary needs.

Why Sample Meal Plans Rock!

Take the guesswork out of eating: No more worrying about what to cook! These plans provide a clear framework with delicious choices.

Discover the power of variety: Explore new foods and taste profiles while keeping your body going.

Fuel your specific needs: Whether you're gluten-free, vegetarian, or simply looking for healthy options, there's a plan for you!

Unleash Your Inner Foodie: Dive into Delicious Diversity!

This chapter goes deep into several sample meal plans, each meant to meet specific dietary preferences:

The Weight-Loss Warrior: This plan focuses on portion control and nutrient-dense meals that keep you feeling full and energetic throughout the day.

The Vegetarian Victory Lap: Plant-powered goodness never tasted so good! Discover how to make vibrant and filling meals packed with protein, healthy fats, and important vitamins.

The Gluten-Free Game Changer: Enjoy great meals without gluten! This plan offers creative replacements and delicious meals that show healthy eating can be a flavor explosion.

The Balanced Bounty: This plan offers a great base for general health and metabolic well-being. It includes a variety of macronutrients and micronutrients to keep your body growing.

Beyond Sample Meals: Building Your Personal Plate!

This part goes beyond just offering pre-made plans. It gives you the information to customize your meals:

Swap and Substitute: Learn how to quickly modify recipes to fit your tastes and dietary restrictions.

Snack Savvy: Discover healthy and satisfying snack choices to keep your energy levels up between meals.

food Prep Magic: Master the art of food prepping to save time and ensure you have healthy options easily available.

Get Ready to Feel the Difference!

By following these sample meal plans and learning how to personalize them, you'll be well on your way to:

Revving up your metabolism: Discover how the right foods can naturally boost your body's fat-burning power.

Unleashing a symphony of flavors: Explore a world of delicious and healthy meals that will tantalize your taste buds.

Embracing lasting change: Learn how to create healthy eating habits that will last a lifetime.

So, what are you waiting for? Turn the page and open a world of delicious options!

Sample Meal Plans for Weight Loss: Ignite Your Metabolism and Blast Fat!

Get ready to ditch the diet yo-yo and accept a sustainable, delicious method of weight loss! This sample meal plan offers exciting takes on classic dishes, focusing on whole foods that fuel your body and fire up your metabolism. Let's get started!

Day 1: The Mediterranean Kickstart

Breakfast (Power Up Your Mornings): Greek Yogurt Power Bowl - Combine 1 cup plain Greek yogurt with 1/4 cup berries, sprinkle with a handful of chopped almonds, and drizzle with 1 tbsp honey.

Lunch (Light & Flavorful): Tuna Niçoise Salad with a Twist - Combine canned tuna, chopped cherry tomatoes, green beans, olives, a hard-boiled egg, and a light vinaigrette sauce. For a protein boost, add beans or lentils.

Dinner (Protein Packed & Satisfying): Salmon with Lemon Herb Crust & Roasted Vegetables - Marinate salmon pieces in lemon juice, olive oil, and your favorite herbs (dill, rosemary, thyme).

Roast alongside bright veggies like broccoli, sweet potato, and carrots.

Day 2: Spice Up Your Life!

Breakfast (Fuel Your Day): Spicy Sweet Potato Scramble - Dice a sweet potato and saute with chopped onion and bell pepper. Scramble 2 eggs with spices like chili powder, cumin, and smoked paprika. Top with salsa and avocado pieces for a smooth kick.

Lunch (On-the-Go Goodness): Turkey and Hummus Wrap - Layer whole wheat pita bread with hummus, sliced turkey, chopped cucumber, and sprouts. Add a spray of sriracha for a touch of heat.

Dinner (Flavorful & Filling): Black Bean Burgers with Chipotle Mayo - Mash black beans with chopped onion, garlic, and spices like cumin and coriander. Form into patties and cook on a pan or grill. Serve on whole-wheat buns with chipotle mayo made with Greek yogurt, lime juice, and adobo sauce.

Day 3: Asian-Inspired Goodness

Breakfast (Quick & Energizing): Tofu Scramble with Vegetables - Crumble tofu and saute with chopped veggies like mushrooms and peppers. Scramble with a splash of soy sauce and olive oil. Add a few sliced green onions on top.

Lunch (Light & Refreshing): Spicy Shrimp and Veggie Noodle Bowl - Saute shrimp with ginger, garlic, and chili flakes. Toss with cooked rice noodles, chopped veggies like carrots and cabbage, and a light soy sauce dressing.

Dinner (Comfort Food with a Twist): Chicken and Broccoli Stir-Fry with Brown Rice - Marinate chicken in soy sauce, ginger, and garlic. Quickly stir-fry with broccoli pieces and serve over brown rice. Finish with a spray of sesame oil and a sprinkle of sesame seeds.

Pro Tip: Throughout the week, snack on fruits, and veggies with hummus, nuts, or a handful of dark chocolate for lasting energy and to avoid cravings. Don't forget to stay refreshed – try for 8 glasses of water per day.

Remember: These are just samples! Feel free to change items based on your tastes and dietary needs. Explore foreign foods and play with new spices to keep your taste buds happy and your metabolism buzzing!

Sample Meal Plans for Maintaining Metabolic Health: Fuel Your Body for Long-Term Vitality

This chapter goes deep into practical meal plans meant to keep your metabolism humming! We'll explore exciting flavor combinations and new products to keep your taste buds happy while supporting your body. Remember, regularity is key, so use these plans as a start to create a personalized approach to healthy eating.

Plan 1: The Mediterranean Marvel

This plan is packed with heart-healthy fats, fiber-rich whole grains, and vibrant veggies – all features of the famous Mediterranean diet.

Breakfast (Power Up Your Morning):

Greek Yogurt Power Bowl: Combine 1 cup plain Greek yogurt with ¼ cup berries, a sprinkle of chopped nuts, and a drizzle of honey.

Lunch (Light & Flavorful):

Tuna Nicoise Salad: Mix canned tuna with chopped cherry tomatoes, Kalamata olives, crumbled feta cheese, a handful of mixed greens, and a light lemon dressing.

Dinner (Flavor Explosion):

Salmon with Roasted Vegetables: Season and bake salmon pieces (4 oz) with lemon slices and fresh herbs. Roast a variety of colorful veggies (broccoli, peppers, onions) with a tablespoon of olive oil and your favorite spices.

Snacks (Bite-Sized Goodness):

Sliced cucumber with hummus

Apple pieces with almond butter

Handful of different nuts and dried fruit

Plan 2: The Spicy Asian Fusion

This plan includes bold flavors and lean protein sources to keep your metabolism wandering and your taste buds tingling.

Breakfast (Savory Start):

Spicy Shrimp Scramble: Sauté chopped shrimp with garlic, ginger, and a pinch of red pepper flakes. Scramble 2 eggs with chopped veggies (onions, peppers) and add the cooked shrimp. Finish with a sprinkling of chopped green onions.

Lunch (Light & Satisfying):

Chicken Lettuce Wraps: Shred cooked chicken breast and toss with a delicious stir-fry sauce (soy sauce, honey, rice vinegar, ginger, garlic).

Fill lettuce leaves with the mixture and top with chopped carrots and onions.

Dinner (Flavorful & Filling):

Black Bean Burgers with Sweet Potato Fries: Make fresh black bean burgers with mashed black beans, breadcrumbs, spices, and an egg. Bake sweet potato fries tossed with olive oil and cinnamon for a sweet-and-salty twist.

Snacks (Sweet & Energizing):

Edamame pods with a sprinkle of sea salt

Cottage cheese with sliced mango

Rice cake with a dollop of natural peanut butter and sliced banana

Beyond the Basics: Spice Up Your Meals

Experiment with Herbs & Spices: Move beyond salt and pepper! Explore herbs like rosemary, thyme, and basil for spicy recipes. Use spices like turmeric, cumin, and chili powder for extra taste and possible health benefits.

Embrace Ethnic Flavors: Get bold and experience the foods of different countries. Korean kimchi, Indian curries, or Thai stir-fries offer bold tastes and a healthy take on your normal meals.

Power Up with Ancient Grains: Incorporate ancient grains like quinoa, brown rice, or barley into your diet. These offer a more complex taste profile and extra nutrients compared to white bread or pasta.

Remember: These are just samples! Feel free to mix and match recipes from both plans, change portion sizes based on your needs, and explore new ingredients to keep your meals interesting and your metabolism thriving!

Chapter 12: Building Sustainable Habits for Long-Term Success: Unlock Your Body's Fat-Burning Code!

Congratulations! You've navigated the exciting world of metabolism, learned how to eat smart, and found strategies to ignite your body's natural fat-burning potential. But the real magic happens now – transforming this discovered information into sustainable habits that strengthen you for life.

This isn't about a quick fix, it's about a living change! Buckle up, because in this chapter, we'll crack the code on building habits that stick. We'll explore the psychology of behavior change, unlock the power of positive feedback, and build a personalized plan for your sustainable success.

Forget the willpower battle! We'll introduce science-backed methods to:

Reprogram Your Mindset: Ditch the self-doubt and develop an optimistic, "I can do this!"

attitude. Learn how to reframe obstacles as chances for growth.

Outsmart Cravings: Discover how to spot your triggers and develop healthy coping methods to silence those pesky cravings before they derail your progress.

Habit building: Unleash the power of habit building! We'll show you how to piggyback healthy habits onto current routines, making them effortless to adopt.

The Power of Small Wins: Celebrate every milestone, no matter how small. We'll study the science behind positive reinforcement and how to use it to fuel your drive.

Building Your Support System: Surround yourself with champions! Learn how to leverage the power of a supportive group to stay accountable and inspired.

This chapter is your unique tool for building a lasting, healthy lifestyle you'll enjoy. We'll provide engaging tasks, self-coaching prompts, and practical tips to build a plan that works for YOU. Imagine waking up each day energized, confident, and in control of your health – that's the power of lasting habits!

Are you ready to open your body's fat-burning code and build a healthier, happier you? Let's dive in!

Unleash Your Inner Powerhouse: Developing a Positive Mindset Around Food and Exercise

Tired of feeling bad about what you eat or fearing your next workout?

It's time to quit the negativity and change your relationship with food and exercise! This guide will be your path to building a positive mindset that feeds your body and ignites your journey to a healthier, happier you.

Get ready to:

Unmask the myths: We'll debunk common misunderstandings about food and exercise that hold you back.

Discover the power of "why": Learn how to tap into your inner reasons for a healthier living.

Celebrate growth, not perfection: Say goodbye to all-or-nothing thoughts and accept a healthy approach.

Transform self-talk: Learn how to quiet your inner critic and become your own biggest fan.

Fuel your body with joy: Explore the delicious world of healthy food that feeds you from the inside out.

Find the movement that excites you: Discover workout routines that are fun, not a job!

This isn't just another diet or workout plan – it's a mental change that will empower you to take control of your health and well-being. Get ready to:

Boost your confidence: Feel great in your own skin as you see and feel the positive changes.

Unleash your inner athlete: Discover the secret power and energy you possess.

Embrace a life of vitality: Experience the joy of moving and the power of good food.

Packed with useful tips, inspiring stories, and engaging tasks, this guide will be your companion on your path to creating a positive mindset and a healthier, happy you!

Are you ready to unlock your full potential? Let's begin your trip today!

Conquer Your Weight Loss Journey: Building a Dream Team for Success!

Tired of going it alone?

Shedding pounds can feel like a hard fight, especially when you're surrounded by temptation and facing plateaus. But what if you had a strong support system cheering you on every step of the way? This chapter is your guide to building a dream team that will inspire you, hold you accountable, and enjoy your wins as you transform your body and life.

Get Ready to:

Unleash the Power of Positive People: Discover the science behind social support and how the right people can skyrocket your success. Learn how to find cheerleaders, accountability partners, and teachers who will feed your drive.

Forge Alliances Beyond the Gym: This isn't just about gym friends! We'll study how to build a support network that includes your family, friends, and even your doctor. Learn strategies to beat possible negativity and enlist them as partners in your weight loss goal.

Embrace the Power of Community: Dive into the exciting world of online communities and support groups. We'll show you how to find like-minded people who share your struggles and successes, giving you a virtual place for encouragement and shared experiences.

Fuel Your Fire with Inspiration: Unlock the power of inspiring stories, podcasts, and social media accounts committed to healthy living. Learn how to create a positive online environment that will keep you motivated and focused on your goals.

Turn Setbacks into Stepping Stones: We'll prepare you with the tools to handle those inevitable bumps in the road. Learn how your support system can help you bounce back from setbacks stronger than ever and keep a positive mindset.

This chapter is your roadmap to building a powerful and helpful network that will inspire you to achieve your weight loss goals and create a permanent lifestyle change. Imagine the difference when you have a team cheering you on, celebrating your victories, and helping you face obstacles. Get ready to change your journey from a solo fight to a successful team effort!

Chapter 13: Conclusion: Embracing a Lifestyle of Health and Vitality

Congratulations! You've reached the final part of your amazing journey toward a revitalized metabolism and a life brimming with energy. Imagine waking up each morning feeling invigorated, your body a highly tuned machine ready to face the day.Imagine clothes fitting easily, your energy rising, and fresh confidence radiating from within.

This, my friend, is the power of accepting a lifestyle of health and energy.

The Spark Has Been Ignited

Throughout this book, we've dug into the fascinating world of metabolism, the engine that drives every function in your body. We've shattered myths about "slow metabolisms" and provided you with the information to improve this powerhouse within. You've learned the power of macronutrients, found how protein fuels your metabolism, and explored the world of healthy fats – important partners, not villains, on your path to health. We've strategized to create calorie gaps, planned to kickstart weight loss, and studied the dynamic duo of exercise and sleep that work synergistically to keep your metabolism humming.

But the Journey Continues...

Think of this book as the starting key. You've turned it, and the engine has roared to life, but the real excitement lies on the open road ahead. The key to long-term success lies in building lasting habits – actions you can weave into the fabric of your daily life.

Building Your Personalized Roadmap

The beauty lies in custom. What works for one individual may not be suitable for another. Experiment with the tactics explained in this book, find what connects with your body and tastes, and create your own path to health.

Fueling Your Body, Nourishing Your Mind

Remember, this trip is not just about physical change. It's about developing a good relationship with food, one built on respect and nourishment. When you favor whole, unprocessed foods, you're giving a message of self-love to your body. Fueling your body with the right nutrients not only aids weight control but also impacts your mental clarity, attention, and happiness.

Celebrate Every Milestone

This trip is a marathon, not a sprint. Celebrate every milestone, every pound lost, every extra mile achieved. Recognize your progress, no matter how modest it may appear. These wins fuel your motivation and keep you going forward.

Embrace the Power of Community

Surround yourself with good forces. Find a helpful community – a friend, a workout buddy, or an online group – who understands your goals and celebrates your successes. Sharing your journey with others strengthens your determination and creates a network of support.

The Greatest Reward: A Life Transformed

The true reward of this trip comes not just in the number on the scale, but in the transformation of your entire life. Imagine a life filled with boundless energy, confidence that radiates from within, and the freedom to follow your interests with gusto. This is the life that awaits you when you adopt a lifestyle of health and energy.

So, what are you waiting for? Step onto the path less traveled, the road that leads to a healthier, happier, and more energetic you. Take the information you've gained, personalize your method, and start creating the life you deserve. Remember, the only boundary is the one you set for yourself. Embrace the adventure and let your light shine!

This book is just the beginning. Now it's your turn to write the next story. Go forth and conquer!.

If this book was enjoyable, please write a review.

Glossary - Unlock the Secrets to Burning Fat!

Welcome to your personal decoder ring for the interesting world of metabolism! This glossary isn't your average dry list of meanings. We're here to make learning these terms fun, and informative, and empower you to become a true metabolism master.

Get ready to:

Blast through jargon: Forget confusing science words! We'll break them down into easy-to-understand bites.

Unlock secret knowledge: Learn the "why" behind the "what" - how these terms impact your weight loss journey and general health.

Become a conversation starter: Impress your friends and family with your increased knowledge of metabolism!

Now, let's dive into the exciting world of terms that will change your understanding of burning fat and achieving lasting health!

Key Terms:

Basal Metabolic Rate (BMR): Think of this as your body's engine idle. It's the number of calories you burn just to stay living (breathing, thinking, etc.). Let's unlock ways to improve your BMR and turn up the fat-burning power!

Calories: Not all calories are made equal! We'll explore the difference between good and bad calories, and how to make smart choices to feed your body for success.

Carbohydrates: Carbs get a bad rap, but they're not all baddies! Learn how to choose the "good carbs" that keep you active and support your metabolism.

Glycemic Index (GI): Ever felt that post-lunch energy crash? The GI explains how different carbs affect your blood sugar, and we'll show you how to choose low-GI options for extended energy and weight control.

Macronutrients: These are the building blocks of your diet: carbs, protein, and fat. We'll study their roles in metabolism and teach you how to make a balanced plate for the best health.

Metabolism: Your body's amazing engine! We'll break down the science behind this process and show you how to improve it for efficient calorie burning.

Micronutrients: Don't let their size fool you! Vitamins and minerals are essential for a healthy body. We'll highlight key elements and how to ensure you get enough.

Protein: The building block of muscle! Discover how protein boosts your metabolism, keeps you feeling fuller for longer, and helps you build a strong, healthy body.

Thermic Effect of Food (TEF): Did you know that just eating burns calories? We'll explain how TEF works and which foods have the best TEF to maximize your calorie-burning ability.

This is just a taste of the exciting terms you'll beat in this dictionary! Remember, information is power. With this glossary as your guide, you'll be well on your way to discovering the secrets of your metabolism and meeting your health and weight loss goals!

I appreciate you journeying with me through each and every page of my book! Your commitment is greatly appreciated.

As a thank you, scan the QR code above to get your unique free gift. Together, let's continue on this incredible adventure.